FIRST AID
WHAT TO DO
IN AN EMERGENCY

by

Robert E. Rothenberg, M.D., F.A.C.S.

D1478098

A Medbook Publication

Published
by

Crown Publishers, Inc.
One Park Avenue
New York, N.Y. 10016

Published simultaneously in Canada by General Publishing Company Limited

First Edition

Printed in the United States of America

Library of Congress Catalog Card Number 76-22832

Excerpts from THE NEW ILLUSTRATED MEDICAL ENCYCLOPEDIA FOR HOME USE used by permission of Harry N. Abrams, Inc.

Exerpts from NEW AMERICAN MEDICAL DICTIONARY AND HEALTH MANUAL used by permission of Crown Publishers, Inc.

CONTENTS

INTRODUCTION

At one time or another, everyone is called upon to render first aid in an emergency. Unless he has taken courses in the subject, there is usually considerable doubt as to what should be done. Some are fearful that they will harm rather than help the victim; others, though well-meaning, through overly energetic maneuvers may actually complicate the situation.

Experience has shown that in the great majority of emergencies, it is better for the uninformed layman to do too little than too much! This dictum is particularly applicable in urban and suburban areas where expert medical help is never more than minutes away.

Some good general rules regarding the giving of first aid are:

1. If expert medical aid is in the immediate vicinity, it is far better to leave the scene of the emergency to fetch help than to attempt to act the role of a professional.

2. If the emergency takes place in an urban area, remember that police and firemen are well trained in first aid and can do more to help than an untrained or partially

trained first-aider.

3. If the emergency takes place in a rural area, remember that there are usually police road patrols available. Ask the first passerby to summon them.

4. Ask the whereabouts of the nearest hospital, and if it is nearby, dispatch someone to notify them that help is needed.

5. In every community, telephone operators know how to obtain help in the quickest way. Tell them the problem and let them follow it up with the proper agencies.

6. Never forget that great physical damage can result from unnecessarily moving the victim of an accident. Of course, if he is pinned under a heavy object or cannot breathe, every attempt should be made to free him. However, it is always better to move the offending object away from the injured person than to attempt to tug and pull the individual from his confined position.

7. Remember that the safest position for an injured person is to lie flat on the floor or ground with his chin up and the collar, tie, and belt loosened. Do not lift up a patient to a sitting, semisitting, or standing position. Do not give him a cigarette, water, whiskey, or anything else to drink, even if he asks for it.

8. Many people who are prone to fainting

spells, seizures, diabetic shock, or convulsions, carry specific instructions in their clothing, wallets, or handbags. If an individual is found unconscious, search his or her apparel for this information.

9. It is a good idea to carry a first-aid guide in the glove compartment of the car. It should be consulted whenever the opportunity presents itself to help someone in need.

10. It is a good idea to carry a ready-made first-aid kit in the glove compartment or trunk of the family car. Or, if one is on any kind of trip that might land him in a place where emergency medical attention might not be immediately available, it is wise to have a first-aid kit in one's suitcase. The kit should contain the following items:

1. Roll of two-inch gauze bandage.
2. Roll of three-inch gauze bandage.
3. Small box of absorbent cotton.
4. Roll of two-inch adhesive tape.
5. Box of Band-Aids.
6. Small box of 3 x 3-inch gauze pads.
7. Box of cotton-tipped applicators.
8. Gauze sling.
9. Six gauze eye pads.
10. Wooden arm splint.
11. Six wooden tongue depressors.

12. Tweezer.
13. Bandage scissors.
14. Small bottle of 70-percent alcohol to be used as a disinfectant.
15. Tube of antibiotic ointment.
16. Small tube of antibiotic eye ointment.
17. Aromatic spirits of ammonia.
18. Six paper cups.
19. Box of toilet tissue.
20. Small bottle of hydrogen peroxide.
21. Box of salt tablets.

1. First-Aid Procedures

ANTIDOTES AND EMERGENCY PROCEDURES FOR POISONING

Many household products and medications, although not true poisons, may be very dangerous if taken internally. It is extremely important to always take special precautions to keep these items out of a child's reach. Every item in the medicine chest must be plainly labeled. This can be done easily by attaching a piece of adhesive tape to the container and writing the name in large letters. *See also THE HOME MEDICINE CHEST.*

All first-aid measures are essentially only emergency measures—UNTIL the doctor arrives. Therefore, if at all possible, it is best to have one person begin the first aid while somebody else summons a doctor. When a doctor is not available, call the police for help.

For GAS POISONING, good rules in an emergency are:

1. Provide fresh air—open all doors and windows and bring the person to the fresh air. Be careful that there is a minimum of exertion on his part.
2. Prevent chilling.
3. Loosen all tight clothing, belts, collars, etc.
4. Keep the person as quiet as possible.
5. Do NOT give alcohol in any form.
6. If the person is unconscious or has stopped breathing, apply artificial respiration.

For SWALLOWED POISONS, good rules in an emergency are:
1. Find the poison container. Most containers of poisonous substances have printed directions pasted on them.
2. If the poisoned person is fully

conscious, induce vomiting.* This should be done only when the person is not in a stuporous condition and there are no convulsions. Also, make sure that the poison swallowed is not a corrosive substance such as kerosene, gasoline, etc.

3. When vomiting and retching begin, place the person face down, with head lower than the rest of the body, so that the vomit will not enter the lungs and cause further damage.

4. Save the poison container, or some of the vomit, for the doctor's inspection. This may help him to decide on the appropriate treatment.

Substances	Procedures
Acids Sulfuric Nitric Hydrochloric Chromic Carbolic	1. Cause vomiting.* 2. Give milk, raw eggs, jello, gelatin. 3. Gargle with solution of bicarbonate of soda.

*To cause vomiting: 1. Add baking soda or salt to drinking water. 2. Give large quantities of warm water. 3. Put finger in back of throat and tickle.

Substances	Procedures
Alcohol	1. Cause vomiting.* 2. Have stomach washed out, preferably at hospital. 3. Keep body warm. 4. Give several cups of black coffee.
Alkalies	1. Give vinegar diluted in water, wine, lemon or apple juice. 2. Cause vomiting. 3. Have stomach washed out as soon as possible. 4. Give milk.
Ammonia	1. Inhale hot vapors. 2. Inhale a dilute vinegar solution.
Arsenic	1. Cause vomiting. 2. Have stomach washed out at nearest hospital. 3. Give milk.
Barbiturates Phenobarbital	1. Cause vomiting 2. Have stomach thoroughly

*To cause vomiting: 1. Add baking soda or salt to drinking water. 2. Give large quantities of warm water. 3. Put finger in back of throat and tickle.

Substances	Procedures
Seconal **Amytal** **Luminal, etc.**	washed out as soon as possible. 3. Apply artificial respiration. † 4. Give laxative. 5. Give strong coffee.
Belladonna *(Atropine)*	1. Cause vomiting. 2. Give strong coffee. 3. Give charcoal tablets. 4. Sponge body with cold water.
Benzine	1. Cause vomiting. 2. Have stomach washed out. 3. Give milk.
Botulism *(and other food poisoning)*	1. Cause vomiting. 2. Have stomach washed out as soon as possible. 3. Give enema with soap suds and water. 4. Give large dose of castor oil. 5. Give charcoal tablets.

†For artificial respiration method, *see* Artificial Respiration.

Substances	Procedures
Bromides	1. Give strong coffee. 2. Have stomach washed out.
Carbon monoxide *(or stove gas)*	1. Take patient to fresh air. 2. Apply artificial respiration. 3. Call police or fire department for oxygen. 4. Keep person lying down and quiet. 5. Keep person warm.
Carbon tetrachloride	1. Apply artificial respiration, if breathing is poor. 2. Have stomach washed out. 3. Give strong coffee.
Chloral hydrate	1. Give oxygen. 2. Apply artificial respiration. 3. Give black coffee, strong. 4. Sponge head with cold water.
Chlorine gas	1. Inhale warm steam. 2. Breathe weak ammonia fumes.
Chloroform	*See* Narcotic poisoning.

Substances	Procedures
Cocaine	1. Cause vomiting.* 2. Have stomach washed out. 3. Apply artificial respiration, if necessary. 4. Give any available barbiturate such as phenobarbital, amytal, etc.
Copper	1. Cause vomiting. 2. Have stomach washed out. 3. Give white of egg every 4 hours. 4. Give charcoal tablets. 5. Give milk.
Corrosive sublimate	*See* Mercury poisoning.
Cyanide	1. Cause vomiting. 2. Have stomach washed out as soon as possible. 3. Apply artificial respiration. 4. Obtain oxygen from police or fire department as soon as possible. 5. Give strong coffee.

*To cause vomiting: 1. Add baking soda or salt to drinking water. 2. Give large quantities of warm water. 3. Put finger in back of throat and tickle.

Substance	Procedures
Digitalis	1. Cause vomiting 2. Give charcoal tablets. 3. Give small doses of alcoholic beverage. 4. Give tea or coffee. 5. Rest in bed.
Ether	*See* Narcotic poisoning.
Illuminating gas	*See* Carbon monoxide poisoning.
Insulin	1. Give sugar or any available candy. 2. Give orange or grape juice.
Iodine	1. Cause vomiting. 2. Have stomach washed out. 3. Give flour or starch in a paste or solution. 4. Give white of raw egg. 5. Give milk. 6. Give bicarbonate of soda solution. 7. Give laxative.
Kerosene	1. Cause vomiting. 2. Have stomach washed out. 3. Give milk.

Substances	Procedures
Lead	1. Cause vomiting.* 2. Have stomach washed out as soon as possible. 3. Give dose of epsom salts. 4. Give white of raw egg and milk. 5. Give charcoal tablets.
Lysol	1. Cause vomiting. 2. Give milk. 3. Give raw eggs, jello, gelatin. 4. Gargle with solution of bicarbonate of soda.
Meat poisoning	1. Cause vomiting. 2. Have stomach washed out as soon as possible. 3. Give enema with soap suds and water. 4. Give large dose of castor oil. 5. Give charcoal tablets.
Mercury	1. Wash out the mouth with sodium perborate solution or other available mouth wash. 2. Cause vomiting.

*To cause vomiting: 1. Add baking soda or salt to drinking water. 2. Give large quantities of warm water. 3. Put finger in back of throat and tickle.

Substance	Procedures
	3. Have stomach washed out as soon as possible.
	4. Give white of eggs and milk.
	5. Give sugar.
	6. Give bicarbonate of soda.
Methyl alcohol	*See* Wood alcohol poisoning.
Morphine	1. Cause vomiting.
	2. Have stomach washed out.
	3. Give strong tea or coffee.
	4. Give charcoal tablets.
	5. Apply artificial respiration.†
Mushrooms	1. Cause vomiting.
	2. Have stomach washed out as soon as possible.
	3. Give starch or flour paste.
	4. Give charcoal tablets.
	5. Give strong tea.
Narcotics	1. Apply artificial respiration.
	2. Cause vomiting.
	3. Give strong coffee or tea.
	4. Give charcoal tablets.

†For artificial respiration method, *see* Artificial Respiration.

Substance	Procedures
Nicotine	1. Have stomach washed out. 2. Give any sedative medication available. 3. Give charcoal tablets.
Opium	*See* Morphine poisoning.
Phenol	*See* Acid poisoning.
Phosphorus	1. Cause vomiting. 2. Have stomach washed out as soon as possible. 3. Give large dose of epsom salts. 4. Give dose of bicarbonate of soda. 5. Do *NOT* give milk or eggs.
Poison ivy or Poison oak	1. Wash thoroughly with soap and water immediately after contact. 2. Wash with rubbing alcohol to relieve itching.
Snake bite	1. Immediate sucking out of wound. 2. Crisscross incision with knife in area of bite. 3. Place tourniquet above the site of the bite. Release every

Substances	Procedures
	20 minutes for a few minutes in order to permit some circulation to return.
	4. Keep patient as quiet and still as possible.
Strychnine	1. Cause vomiting.
	2. Have stomach washed out as soon as possible.
	3. Give any sedative available.
	4. Give moderate dose of alcoholic beverage.
	5. Apply artificial respiration if breathing is poor.†
Sulfur	1. Apply artificial respiration.
	2. Give salt water to drink.
Tobacco	*See* Nicotine poisoning.
Wood alcohol *(methyl alcohol)*	1. Cause vomiting.
	2. Have stomach washed out.
	3. Keep body warm.
	4. Apply artificial respiration if necessary.
	5. Give strong coffee.
Zinc	1. Cause vomiting.
	2. Have stomach washed out.
	3. Give white of egg and milk.
	4. Give strong tea.

†For artificial respiration method, *see* Artificial Respiration.

2. Artificial Respiration
(Mouth-to-Mouth Method)

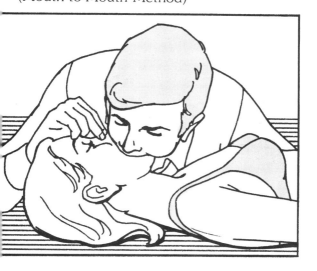

a. Apply in all cases where breathing has stopped—whether due to drowning, suffocation, poisoning, etc.
b. Stretch out patient on his back; loosen any tight clothing around the neck or chest.
c. Lift up chin and tilt head back as far as possible. (This straightens out the windpipe and improves the airway to the lungs.)

d. With your fingers, pinch the patient's nostrils so that they are closed.

e. Place your mouth tightly over patient's mouth and blow as hard as you can.

f. Take your mouth away to permit air to be expelled from the lungs.

g. Repeat this every 5-6 seconds.

h. Continue this maneuver so long as there is any pulse or heartbeat. It may take several hours to revive someone.

i. When you tire, have someone substitute for you.

j. If the patient seems to have water or mucus in his throat or chest, tilt him upside down or on his side to permit such fluid to run out the mouth.

k. Wipe out patient's mouth with your fingers if mucus or other material collects there. (A nonbreathing person will never bite.)

l. If you are squeamish about direct mouth-to-mouth contact, you may blow through an opened handkerchief. (This may not prove to be as effective as direct contact.)

m. Discontinue artificial respiration only when you are certain there is no pulse or heartbeat for several minutes. Listen carefully with your ear to patient's left chest region.

n. If patient is revived, keep him warm and do not move him until the doctor arrives, or at least for one-half hour.

3. Bites

A. Animal or Human Bites

1. Scrub wound thoroughly for 5-10 minutes with a mild soap and plenty of warm water.
2. Apply a sterile gauze bandage, or if this is not available, use a clean handkerchief.
3. Take patient to a doctor who may give tetanus antitoxin, tetanus toxoid, or, possibly, antibiotics. If the bite has been caused by a dog, cat, rat, or other animal, your physician may recommend antirabies injections.
4. Do *NOT* pour strong antiseptics, such as iodine, on a wound caused by a bite.
5. If possible, catch the animal causing the bite, and turn him over to a veterinarian to see if he has rabies.

B. Insect Bites

1. If a sting has been left in place, such as with a bee, wasp, etc., pluck it out. Do so gently, in order to avoid breaking the sting.

2. If a great deal of swelling is present, this indicates a marked sensitivity to the bite poison. In such cases, place a tourniquet above the bite area so that the poison will be more slowly absorbed. Loosen the tourniquet every 10 to 15 minutes to permit return of circulation.

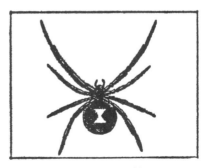

Black widow spider

3. If the bite is caused by an insect which burrows under the skin, such as a chigger, or by one which attaches itself to the skin, such as a tick, wash the area thoroughly with soap and water. A drop or two of turpentine may dislodge a tick or kill a chigger. Cover with Vaseline so that the insect cannot breathe.

4. Antiallergic (antihistamine) medications may be prescribed by your physician to reduce the swelling and itching.

5. Do *NOT* scratch a bite area as it may lead to greater absorption of the poison or to infection.

6. If the bite has been caused by a black widow spider, treat as a snake bite.

C. Snake Bites

1. Treat all snake bites as if they have been caused by poisonous snakes, unless you are thoroughly familiar with the various types of snakes.

2. A tourniquet should be placed above the site of the bite. Do this immediately.

3. Crossed incisions *through* the skin should be made over the two fang marks. A penknife may be used. Do not

wait to sterilize it. The incisions should be ¼ inch long.

4. The bite should be sucked out thoroughly. (No harm can come from swallowing, or taking into the mouth, the venom of a poisonous snake.)

5. The tourniquet should be loosened every 15 minutes for 2-3 minutes and then reapplied.

6. Suction to the wound should be repeated every 5 minutes for an hour.

7. Have victim lie down and keep quiet, so as to reduce circulation.

8. If ice, or running cold water, is available immerse the bitten area so as to reduce circulation.

9. Take victim to nearest hospital so that the appropriate antivenin can be administered.

10. If possible, kill the snake and take it to the hospital so that it can be identified. (Antivenin is effective only for the specific type of snake causing the bite.)

4. Bleeding
(Hemorrhage)

a. Have patient lie down flat.

b. Place sterile gauze pad, sanitary napkin, clean handkerchief, etc., directly over the wound.

c. Apply direct, firm pressure (with your fingers or hand) over the wound; continue pressure for 5-15 minutes.

d. If bleeding does not stop with prolonged direct pressure, and the wound is in the arm or leg, apply a tourniquet for 10-15 minutes. Release to see if bleeding has stopped. If not, reapply tourniquet and transport patient to nearest doctor.

e. Do *NOT* apply a tourniquet until you have first tried pressure upon arteries supplying the arm and leg. This will often stop the bleeding and make the use of a tourniquet unnecessary. (These pressure points are located on the inner side of the upper arm and just below the groin.)

f. Most bleeding, unless from a major vessel, will stop within a few minutes. Clean wound thoroughly with plain soap and water. If bleeding is too active, apply a tourniquet for 10 minutes in order to thoroughly cleanse the wound.

g. Bandage to stop bleeding should *NOT* be applied so tightly that it will interfere with circulation. If the patient feels it is too tight, or if the tissue below the bandage swells or turns blue in color, cut the bandage down the middle and apply new bandage material more loosely *over* the original bandage.

h. Take patient to doctor for possible further cleansing and stitching of the wound.

i. Internal bleeding will usually evidence itself by the coughing up or vomiting of blood or "coffee ground" appearing material. Bleeding from the urinary tract will show itself upon passage of bloody urine. Bleeding from the intestinal tract will show itself by blood in the stool or by passage of black, tarry stools. Have such a patient:

    1. Lie flat.
    2. Breathe deeply.
    3. Transport him as soon as possible to a hospital.
    4. Do *NOT* attempt to give medicines to such patients.

j. Bleeding from areas where tourniquets cannot be applied, such as the neck, should be treated by applying direct finger pressure over the wound. Keep pressure in place until doctor arrives.

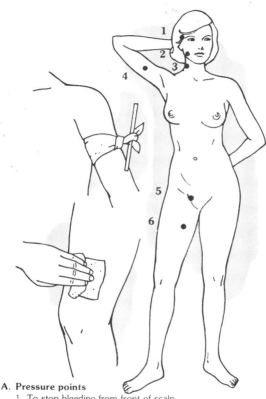

A. Pressure points
1. To stop bleeding from front of scalp
2. To stop bleeding from face
3. To stop jugular vein bleeding
4. To stop bleeding from arm and hand
5. To stop bleeding from thigh and leg
6. To stop bleeding from leg

B. Tourniquet applied to stop bleeding from arm and hand

C. Diagram showing direct pressure to stop local bleeding

5. Burns

a. *First-degree burns* extend only to the top layers of the skin. They can usually be self-treated by applying plain Vaseline or any other mild ointment which soothes the reddened area and prevents the skin from becoming too dry. (Sunburn, without blister formation, is the most common type of first-degree burn.)

b. *Second-degree burns* extend deeper into the skin than first-degree burns but do not involve the very deepest layer, the corium. They can be diagnosed by noting blisters and destruction of the top layers of skin.

> 1. Such burned areas should be immediately placed under cold running water for 10-15 minutes and, if dirty, mild (soap) cleansing should be carried out.
> 2. A clean, sterile gauze dressing should be applied.
> 3. The patient should drink large quantities of fluids.
> 4. Blisters should *NOT* be opened.
> 5. The patient should be taken to a physician for further treatment.

c. *Third- and Fourth degree burns* extend to or through all the layers of the skin. First aid should include:

1. Place area under cold, running water.
2. Gently clean away dirt. If clothes can be removed from the burned area without pulling away tissue, this should be done.
3. Do *NOT* put butter or ointments on deep burned areas.
4. Patients should be given large quantities of fluids.
5. If patient is in shock, he should be covered with blanket and transported, on a stretcher, to the nearest hospital.

d. *Chemical burns* should be immediately flushed with cold running water to wash away the chemical. Cover the burned area with a sterile dressing. Patient should then be taken to a doctor.
e. *Eye burns* should be flushed with large amounts of water. The eye should then be covered with a sterile dressing and the patient taken to a physician.

6. Carbon monoxide (gas) poisoning

Carbon monoxide gas has no odor. It may originate from the exhaust of an automobile, or from defective stoves burning wood, coal or oil, etc.

   a. Open all windows and doors to permit fresh air into the area.
   b. Start artificial respiration if the patient is not breathing spontaneously or regularly. Continue as long as the heart is beating.
   c. Encourage deep breathing of fresh air.
   d. Keep patient lying down quietly.
   e. Keep patient warm.
   f. Notify the police or fire department, who will respond with emergency equipment.

7. Cardiac Arrest and Cardiac Massage.

Cardiac arrest means heart stoppage. It may be caused by a heart attack, a severe electric shock, or as a result of a pulmonary embolus, or it may occur during anesthesia or an operation. Whatever its cause, cardiac arrest means that the heart has abruptly stopped beating.

Cardiac arrest can be diagnosed readily by placing one's ear on the left chest and noting if there is a heartbeat. This is a much more accurate method of determining cardiac arrest than taking the pulse. In some instances, the heartbeat may be so weak as not to be transmitted to the wrist.

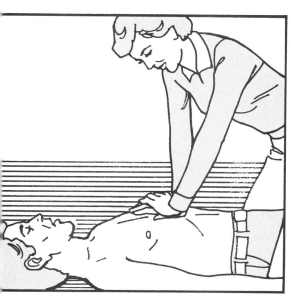

Closed method of cardiac massage

Here is the way to carry out cardiac massage:

1. Place patient flat on his back on a hard surface.
2. If patient is in bed, lift him to the floor.
3. Kneel and straddle the patient.
4. Place the heel of the palm of the right hand on victim's breastbone.
5. Place the left hand over the right hand and push down so that the breastbone is depressed about one to two inches.
6. Release the pressure of your hands.
7. Repeat this maneuver every 1 to 2 seconds 15 times.
8. Stop the cardiac massage briefly in order to give mouth-to-mouth artificial respiration for 2 to 3 breaths. (Remember, a person whose heart has stopped will not breathe spontaneously.)
9. Resume the cardiac massage for another 15 strokes. Stop again for mouth-to-mouth breathing.
10. If someone else is available, have him render the mouth-to-mouth artificial respiration at the same time that you are conducting the cardiac massage. In such an instance, the cardiac massage

is continued without stopping after every 15 strokes.

11. Cardiac massage should be continued for at least 15 minutes to make absolutely sure the heart action has stopped completely.

12. Do not depend solely on the pulse to determine if the heart has resumed beating. Stop for a second or two and place your ear against the victim's chest wall.

13. Any flicker of sound, even a faint beat, is an indication to continue the cardiac massage.

14. Do not stop the cardiac massage until the heart has resumed a regular or near-regular beat or until you have determined positively, after 15 minutes, that there are no heartbeats whatever.

15. If the heart has resumed beating and you have discontinued the cardiac massage, send for immediate medical assistance. DO NOT MOVE THE PATIENT. Let him lie quiet until professional help arrives.

CAUTION

Cardiac massage is given only when the

heart has stopped. It is NOT given for unconsciousness, heart attack, shock, drowning, or any other emergency, IF THERE IS A READILY HEARD HEART-BEAT.

34

8. Choking

a. Encourage strenuous coughing. This is often all that is necessary to get rid of the food or foreign body that is causing the choking.
b. If the victim is a child, hold him upside down and slap him sharply on the back.
c. If the obstructing object is not expelled, place index finger in mouth and sweep it around the back of throat. In a child, this usually will cause the foreign body to be dislodged.
d. The newest first-aid method to relieve choking from food or a foreign body in the windpipe involves the following maneuvers:
   1. Raise the victim to his feet.
   2. Get behind him and place both your arms about his waist at a level just below the rib cage.
   3. Place your right fist high up in his abdomen, just below the breastbone.

4. Firmly grasp your right fist with your left hand so that you are now holding him tightly.

5. With a sudden inward and upward thrust, tighten your grip as forcefully as you can. Release pressure immediately. This will cause a tremendous increase of pressure within the victim's chest cavity and will force air, along with the foreign body or food, out of the windpipe.

6. If the first thrust fails to clear the windpipe, repeat it. Remember, the thrust must be an instantaneous one. Do not maintain your tight grip once you have carried out the thrust.

7. This method is reserved for adults. A vigorous thrust in a child might produce internal injuries.

e. If all attempts to relieve the choking by the above methods fail and the victim turns blue and cannot breathe at all, and if a doctor is not available—and only when it is obvious that death will ensue—an emergency tracheotomy may be performed. This is done by stabbing a hole with a knife into the windpipe below the Adam's apple. The hole is kept open, so that air can pass in and out of it, by twisting the knife blade.

f. If the patient is able to breathe but the offending food or foreign body has not been coughed up, it is essential that he be taken to the nearest doctor or hospital. Do this even if the choking has subsided because some foreign bodies, or chunks of food may go deep into the bronchial tubes where they will eventually cause infection.

Cold. See Exposure, Frosbite

9. Convulsions

a. Prevent further self-injury by protecting the patient, particularly the head.
b. Place patient on the floor or ground and give plenty of room for him to thrash about.
c. Loosen clothing around the neck and lift up the chin so that breathing is unobstructed.

d. If possible, place a folded handkerchief between the teeth, to prevent tongue biting. (Keep your own fingers away from patient's teeth, to avoid being accidentally bitten.)

e. Do *NOT* throw cold water on these patients in an attempt to revive them.

f. Do *NOT* try to restrain their convulsive movements.

g. Most convulsions last only a few minutes. After recovery, comfort the patient, keep him quiet, and send for a physician.

Convl

h. Do not leave a patient alone, after he has emerged from a convulsion, for at least one-half hour. (They are often confused and it may take this length of time for them to fully regain their normal mental and physical senses.)

i. Search the patient's clothing for information. Epileptics and diabetics often carry instructions on what should be done for them.

j. Do *NOT* pick up a convulsing child and run for a doctor. It is better to keep him in his own bed.

k. Do *NOT* place a convulsing child in water. Keep him in bed.

10. Dislocations

a. Do *NOT* try to replace a dislocation yourself.

b. If a doctor is nearby, transport patient with as little movement of the joint as possible.

c. If you are a long distance from a hospital or doctor, bind the dislocated limb with a towel, bandage, etc., so that it does not move.

    1. Gently tie dislocated ankle, knee or leg to the normal limb on the other side.

    2. Bind the arm in which there is a dislocation to the chest and abdomen.

d. If neck dislocation is suspected, firmly pull on head and hold it in a straight position without permitting movement.

11. Drowning. See also Artificial Respiration

a. If patient is breathing, place him on his abdomen with head turned to one side.

b. Do *NOT* place over a barrel or attempt to hold upside down. Water from the lungs will be brought up spontaneously if the patient is breathing.

c. If the patient is not breathing, place flat on his *back*, lift up the chin and commence artificial respiration.

d. If mouth-to-mouth breathing does not get air into the lungs, it indicates a severe spasm of the larynx. Continued spasm may require an emergency tracheotomy (*See* Choking) *but if it has to be performed by other than a doctor, it should be done only when it is obvious that the patient is not getting air into the lungs and is dying.*

e. Continue artificial respiration as long as there is any pulse or heartbeat. This may mean hours!

f. Send for doctor, police, or fire department as soon as possible.

12. Electric Shock

a. Do *NOT* touch a person who is still in contact with an electric current. This may electrocute you.

b. Remove electric contact from patient, or the patient from electric contact, as quickly as possible.

1. Use a *dry* stick to shove away wire or to move the patient.
2. Cut off the source of current, such as an electric plug, if this is possible, or
3. Use an axe, with a wooden handle, to chop the wire bearing the current.
4. Do *NOT* attempt to remove a victim from his electric contact unless your body and hands are dry and you are standing on dry ground or on a dry surface.

c. If victim is not breathing, start mouth-to-mouth artificial respiration. Continue so long as there is any pulse or heartbeat.
d. Keep victim warm.
e. Send for doctor, police, or fire department, for additional help in resuscitation.
f. Give first aid to any burned area on body. (*See* Burns)

13. Exposure (Cold). See also Frostbite

a. Wrap patient in blankets.
b. Place in warm room.

c. Place in tub of warm (not too hot) water.

d. Dry body and place in warm bed.

e. Give warm drinks.

f. Do *NOT* give alcoholic beverage.

g. If necessary, start mouth-to-mouth artificial respiration.

14. Fainting, Dizziness, and Vertigo

a. Place patient in a lying-down position with face up and head at body level or slightly lower.

b. Elevate legs to slightly above level of rest of body. (Use pillow, coat, blanket, etc.)

c. Loosen collar or any tight clothing that might interfere with breathing.

d. If breathing is shallow or stops, apply mouth-to-mouth method of artificial respiration.

e. Keep in lying-down position at least 15 minutes after regaining consciousness.

f. Do *NOT* throw cold water in face.

g. Examine head to make sure patient did not injure himself, if he fell during faint.

h. If patient has merely had dizziness, or vertigo, do not permit him to arise until the symptoms have completely disappeared.

i. If the fainting, dizziness, or vertigo persists for more than a few minutes, call a physician.

15. Foreign Bodies

A. Eyes

1. Blink eyelids repeatedly to stimulate flow of tears which may wash out foreign body.
2. Do *NOT* rub eye. (This merely makes foreign body embed itself deeper.)
3. Wash out eye by dropping in drops of lukewarm water.
4. Draw down lower lid. If foreign body is embedded in lower lid, take moistened edge of clean handkerchief and gently wipe it off.
5. Bend up upper lid. If foreign body is embedded in upper lid, take moistened edge of clean handkerchief and gently wipe it off.
6. If foreign body is embedded in

the pupil or in the colored portion of the eye, do NOT try to remove it. See a doctor.

7. If foreign body has been removed, irritation of the eye can be relieved by dropping in a drop or two of mineral oil or castor oil.

B. Ears

1. No lasting harm can come from a foreign body in the ear. Therefore, do NOT get excited or put a sharp instrument into the ear canal.
2. Have patient lie down and pour in sufficient mineral oil, castor oil, or olive oil to fill the canal. Permit it to stay there a few minutes. This will usually float out or dislodge a foreign body.
3. If foreign body does not come out, take patient to a physician.

C. Nose

1. Stimulate sneezing by having patient sniff pepper or by tickling

the opposite nostril. This will
usually dislodge a foreign body.
2. If foreign body is not extruded,
take patient to a physician.

D. *Splinters*

1. Only those splinters which
protrude from the skin surface
should be removed by
nonmedical personnel.
2. Grasp firmly and withdraw
slowly so as not to break.
3. Apply peroxide or alcohol to
area, and cover with sterile
bandage.
4. If splinter breaks off beneath the
skin, take patient to a physician.
Most foreign bodies become
infected if permitted to remain in
place.
5. Do *NOT* try to probe deep into
the skin for a splinter. You may
spread infection or push it
deeper!

E. *Dirt in Cuts or Lacerations*
(See Lacerations, Scrapes, and
Contusions)

F. Swallowed Foreign Bodies

1. Rounded objects such as marbles, nickles, dimes, buttons, etc., usually pass through the intestinal tract without causing any disturbance. Strain the stool daily and note its passage.

2. Open pins, needles, nails, if swallowed, may cause trouble but the majority of them do pass through uneventfully. However, see your doctor. He will X-ray the child and will advise further treatment, if necessary. Strain stool to note passage.

3. Do *NOT* give laxatives to children who have swallowed foreign bodies.

4. Give normal diet.

5. Call physician if child has trouble in breathing or has abdominal pain.

16. Fractures and Severe Sprains

a. If medical aid is available, do *NOT* move the patient or the injured part. Permit *NO* weight-bearing!

Frctr

b. Do *NOT* try to push back a broken bone if it protrudes from the skin.

c. Do *NOT* try to straighten a fracture yourself, if a physician will become available.

d. Keep the patient warm.

e. If patient must be moved. *splint* the broken bones before moving:

    1. An injured collarbone, shoulder, or arm should be splinted by wrapping the arm securely to the body. Do *NOT* bend the arm if it is found in a hanging position. If found with elbow bent, then splint it in that position.

    2. Splint fractured leg in a straight position and then tie it to opposite leg, so as to prevent movement.

    3. A cane, umbrella, straight pieces of wood, etc., can be used as a splint. A torn shirt, or handkerchiefs, can be used as bandage material.

    4. Always pad with something, such as a piece of clothing, between the splint and the injured part of the body.

f. Transport patient in a lying-down

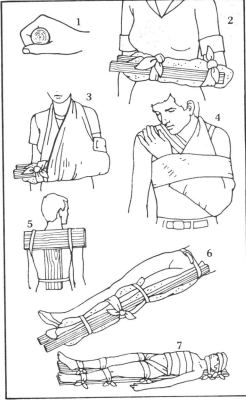

Splints

1. Bandage roll in hand for broken fingers or hand bones (metacarpals)
2. Splints of scrap wood padded with towels for broken forearm
3. Broken forearm supported by a sling
4. Sling and band for broken collarbone or dislocated shoulder
5. "T" board for broken collarbone
6. Splint of scrap wood or tree limbs padded with towels and bound with handkerchiefs and belts
7. Splints for severe back injury or high thigh break or broken pelvis

position. A blanket or overcoat may be used as a stretcher if several people are available to carry the patient.

g. Give the same first aid to a sprain as you would to a fracture. A layman cannot distinguish between a fracture and sprain.

h. Do *NOT* apply a tourniquet to limb unless there is uncontrollable bleeding.

i. If the fracture is accompanied by an open wound, cover such wound with a sterile dressing. If this is not available, use a clean handkerchief.

j. Broken Neck or Back:
   1. Do *NOT* move patient!
   2. Keep body straight.
   3. Do *NOT* lift the head or bend it forward!
   4. Keep patient lying down.
   5. If patient *must* be moved, place on stomach and transport on blanket, with head straight for back injury. Transport face up for neck injury.

17. Frostbite

a. Warm the patient gradually (room temperature).

b. Give warm liquids and food.
c. Thaw out frostbitten parts *slowly*.
d. Give medications to relieve pain (aspirin, etc.).

e. Start moving frostbitten part slowly.
f. Do *NOT:*
    1. Give alcohol to patient.
    2. Immerse frostbitten part in *hot* water.
    3. Rub frostbitten part.
    4. Apply snow.
g. Keep sterile dressing over frostbitten part, as skin may eventually break, leaving an open wound.

Gas Poisoning. See Antidotes and Emergency Procedures for Poisoning, Carbon Monoxide Poisoning; also Artificial Respiration.

18. Head Injuries

a. Have patient lie flat on his back.
b. Keep patient warm.
c. Do not permit patient to get up and walk about.
d. If there has been loss of consciousness, patient should be transported to hospital for further observation.

e. If there is bleeding from an ear, it usually indicates a skull fracture.

f. If there is a cut on the head, apply a sterile dressing or clean handkerchief.

g. Do *Not* give alcohol or any medication to relieve headache. This may mask symptoms.

h. Patient must be advised to consult a physician within the few hours after a head injury. Some injuries appear trivial at first but then develop into serious injuries within twenty-four hours.

i. Fractured Jaw:

    1. Close the mouth so that teeth come together as closely as possible.

    2. Tie a handkerchief or scarf so that it circles the head, from beneath the chin to the top of the head.

    3. Permit patient to remain in a sitting position.

    4. Urge patient not to attempt to move the jaw or to talk.

19. Heart Attacks

Here are first-aid rules in heart attacks.

a. Do not move patient!
b. Keep patient in semi-sitting position.
c. Open collar, loosen tie and belt.
d. Encourage deep breathing.
e. Give patient medication which he may have in the possession (if he has had previous attacks).

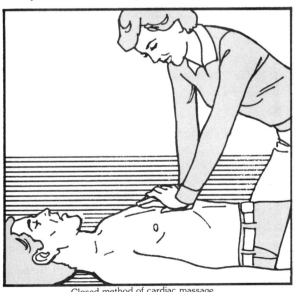

Closed method of cardiac massage

f. If heart stops beating, use "closed method" cardiac massage:

1. Place patient flat on back.
2. Kneel and straddle patient.
3. Place heel of palm of right hand on patient's breastbone.
4. Place left hand over your right hand and push down so that breastbone is depressed about one inch.
5. Release.
6. Repeat this every 1-2 seconds for at least 15 minutes or until heartbeat and breathing are resumed.
7. If someone else is also available, have him render mouth-to-mouth artificial respiration at the same time as you are conducting cardiac massage.

g. Do not permit a patient who has undergone an obvious heart attack to move until he has been examined by a physician. (Pains which have subsided may return with greater intensity if the patient is allowed to exert himself.) Most heart attacks are accompanied by severe vise-like, crushing chest pains beneath the breastbone in the center of the chest. Often, the pain spreads to the left arm and down to the ring finger of the hand.

20. Heat Stroke and Heat Exhaustion

a. Get the victim out of the sun or out of the hot place.
b. Place him in cold water or, if not possible, keep pouring cold water over him.
c. Wrap victim in cold, wet sheets or towels.
d. Give cold water to drink (4-5 glasses.)
e. Give 1/2 teaspoonful of ordinary table salt with water every half hour for 3 to 4 doses.
f. If possible, give the victim an enema with iced water.
g. Do not permit victim to move about.
h. Summon a physician.

Heat

21. Lacerations (Cuts), Scrapes, and Contusions.

a. Before rendering first aid, wash your own hands so that you do not contaminate the victim's cut or scrape.
b. If possible, place the injured part under running, lukewarm water for about 5 minutes.
c. With sterile gauze, absorbent cotton, or

if they are not available, a clean handkerchief, wash out the wound, using a mild soap and warm water.

d. Gently wipe away any dirt or pieces of clothing that have become loose after the washing.

e. A deep scrape (abrasion) or scratch occurring in dirt or cinders must be scrubbed thoroughly to remove all visible dirt particles. This should be carried out, even if painful, in order to avoid subsequent infection or tetanus (lockjaw).

f. Most superficial wounds will stop bleeding spontaneously unless a large blood vessel has been severed. If marked bleeding and spurting continues, apply a tourniquet above the wound, being sure to release it every 15 minutes. Remember that it is always preferable to stop bleeding by direct pressure over the wound. Tourniquets should be applied only as a last resort.

g. Cover wound with sterile gauze or clean handkerchief. Apply direct, steady pressure to stop bleeding.

h. Do *NOT* pour alcohol, iodine, or other

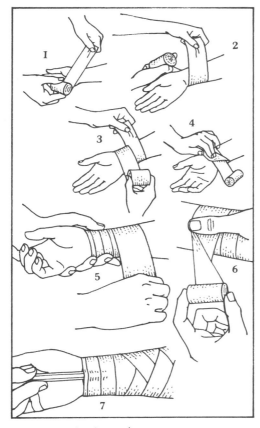

1—4. Steps in the bandage anchor
  5. The roller bandage
  6. Starting the "reverse" for the spiral reverse bandage for regions
     whose diameter changes
  7. Testing for tightness

strong antiseptics on an open wound! Soap and water cleansing is much better as a safeguard against infection!

i. If tissues beneath the skin can be seen through the open wound, it is usually an indication that suturing (stitching) will be necessary. Take patient to a surgeon or nearest physician.

j. It is particularly important to get medical care for cuts and abrasions which originate outdoors, in dirty areas. Such wounds are more prone to infections. Wounds incurred in fields where cattle, horses, etc., are present, should be watched for tetanus. Tetanus antitoxin or toxoid is usually given in cases where wounds have resulted from rusty objects.

k. A severe contusion (bruise) should be treated by the application of steady pressure with the hand over the injured area. Ice or cold water should be applied for 20 minutes at a time, with a similar period of withdrawal of the application. Bruises more than a few hours old can no longer be helped by cold applications. Raise the injured part, such as a leg, to body level so that there will be less tendency for blood to gravitate to the area.

l. Pain, redness, heat, swelling, or pink streaks leading away from a lacerated area are indications that infection has set in. See a doctor!

22. Nosebleed

a. Place patient in a sitting position.

b. Pack the bleeding nostril with a piece of clean absorbent cotton.

c. If there are nosedrops handy, moisten the packing with a few drops as this may help to contract the bleeding vessel.

d. Exert firm finger pressure against the bleeding nostril for at least 10 minutes

Nose

e. Have patient bend head slightly forward during this maneuver. This will prevent blood from trickling down the back of the throat.

f. Leave cotton packing in place for 2—3 hours.

g. If bleeding does not stop, take patient to a doctor who will cauterize the bleeding point.

h. If bleeding is coming from the back part of the nose (only about 10% of cases) the above first aid will not help. Take such people to a physician as soon as possible. Do *NOT* panic; nosebleeds do not cause healthy people to hemorrhage seriously.

i. Do *NOT* place a cold key in the back of the neck. It won't help.

23. Poison Ivy or Poison Oak

a. Wash the skin thoroughly with soap and water immediately after contact.
b. Wash with rubbing alcohol to relieve itching.

24. Radiation Exposure

a. Get out of the radiation area as quickly as possible.
b. Cleanse *all* parts of your body in soap and water. Wash over and over again, for at least one half hour.
c. Discard all clothing, and all other objects, which were with you in an exposed area.
d. Contact the local authorities for further instructions.

25. Shock*

a. Place the patient on his back with his feet at a higher level than his head.

b. If there is active bleeding contributing toward the shock, measures should be taken to stop it. *See also* Bleeding.

c. Keep patient warm but do not overheat.

d. If there is severe pain (one of the greatest causes of shock) medication should be given as soon as possible to relieve it.

e. If there is a fractured bone (a frequent contribution toward shock), it should be splinted and immobilized at once.

f. If it can be ascertained positively that there has been no abdominal injury, and that the cause of the shock does not have anything to do with abdominal organs, then warm fluids may be given.

g. Do *NOT* give alcohol, tea, or coffee!

h. Transport patient in lying-down position to the nearest hospital.

*The diagnosis of shock can be made by noting the following symptoms and signs:
  1. The skin is gray, cold, and sweaty.
  2. There may or may not be loss of consciousness.
  3. Pulse is weak and rapid.
  4. Breathing is rapid and shallow.
  5. Pupils of the eyes are dilated.
  6. Patient is excessively thirsty.
  7. If conscious, patient is apprehensive and frightened.

26. Stab and Puncture Wounds

a. Move the patient as little as possible.
b. If the stabbing object (a knife or pick) can be withdrawn easily, do so. This may prevent further injury to tissues when the patient moves.
c. Note carefully the angle and depth of the stabbing object so that you can report it accurately to the attending physician.
d. If the wound is in the chest, and air is being sucked into and blown out of the chest, cover the opening tightly. It can be plugged best with a sterile gauze dressing and adhesive tape. However, a clean handkerchief, scotch tape, a tie, etc., can also be used to plug the opening.
e. Stop active bleeding. (*See* Bleeding for method)
f. If any internal organs are protruding through the wound, cover them with a sterile gauze dressing or a clean handkerchief.
g. Stab wounds always require expert care. Take patient to a doctor who will, in most instances, give tetanus antitoxin or toxoid.

h. Small puncture wounds should have their edges spread so as to promote some bleeding and prevent the sealing in of dirt, rust, etc.

27. Suffocation or Strangulation. See also Artificial Respiration; Carbon monoxide poisoning; Choking

a. Place patient in open air or throw open all windows.
b. Loosen anything tight around the neck, chest, or abdomen.
c. Lift up the chin to improve airway.
d. Wipe away any secretions which may have collected in the mouth.
e. If foreign body is lodged in the throat, turn patient upside down and strike sharply on the back.
f. Put index finger in mouth and try to sweep out any foreign body which may be stuck in back of throat.
g. Encourage deep breathing and then a forceful cough.
h. Employ mouth-to-mouth breathing as described under Artificial Respiration.
i. Summon police or fire department, who will respond with Pulmotor and oxygen.

Stab

28. Toothache

a. Apply a hot water bag or ice bag to the side of the face, whichever gives more relief.
b. Take aspirin or other pain-relieving medications.
c. Call your dentist. You *will* be able to reach him at night if you try.

29. Unconsciousness. See also Fainting

a. If patient is not breathing but has a pulse or heartbeat, apply mouth-to-mouth breathing.
b. Search the patient's clothing. You may find information that he is a diabetic, epileptic, heart patient, etc.
c. Keep patient lying flat on back with chin up.
d. Loosen tight clothing.
e. Check for possible head injury or bleeding.
f. Summon ambulance by telephoning the police.
g. Give nothing by mouth.
h. Do *NOT* throw cold water in face.
i. Keep patient warm. Cover with coat or

blanket.

j. If patient is convulsing, try to place folded handkerchief between teeth. Be careful that you are not bitten accidentally.

II. Temperature

In determining the condition of any patient, it is important for the first-aider to understand the significance of body temperature, pulse rates, and rates of respiration. Any nurse or doctor will be happy to teach anyone how to read a thermometer and how to take and count the pulse. One needs no instruction on how to count the number of breaths a person takes each minute.

In most illnesses associated with infection, the temperature, pulse, and respiratory rates increase. The more severe the infection, the higher will be temperature, pulse, and respiratory rates.

1. Normal Body Temperature

Children: 99° F.
Adults: 98.6° F.
   a. Rectal thermometer readings tend to be

up to one-half degree more than those recorded by mouth thermometers.
b. Temperatures tend to be lowest on rising in the morning, and may rise as much as one degree toward evening.

2. Centigrade and Fahrenheit Systems

	Centigrade	Fahrenheit
Normal Body Temperature	37.0°	98.6°
Boiling Water (Sea Level)	100.0°	212.0°
Freezing Water (Sea Level)	.0°	32.0°

To convert Fahrenheit to Centigrade: Subtract 32 and multiply by 5/9.
To convert Centigrade to Fahrenheit: Multiply by 9/5 and add 32.

3. Temperature-Pulse Relations

A variation of one degree of temperature above 98° F. is approximately equivalent to a rise of 10 beats in pulse rate, thus:

Temp.	98°F. corresponds with pulse of 60 per minute
	99°F. ,, ,, ,, ,, 70 ,, ,,
	100°F. ,, ,, ,, ,, 80 ,, ,,
	101°F. ,, ,, ,, ,, 90 ,, ,,
	102°F. ,, ,, ,, ,,100 ,, ,,
	103°F. ,, ,, ,, ,,110 ,, ,,
	104°F. ,, ,, ,, ,,120 ,, ,,
	105°F. ,, ,, ,, ,,130 ,, ,,

Comparative Temperature Scales

CENTIGRADE	FAHRENHEIT
	220
100	210
	200
90	190
	180
80	170
70	160
	150
60	140
	130
50	120
	110
40	100
	90
30	80
20	70
	60
10	50
	40
0	30
	20
10	10
	0
20	10

Temp

III. Pulse Rates

	Average Beats per Minute
The Unborn Child	140 to 150
Newborn Infants	130 to 140
During first year	110 to 130
During second year	96 to 115
During third year	86 to 105
7th to 14 year	76 to 90
14th to 21st year	76 to 85
21st to 60th year	70 to 75
After 60th year	67 to 80

1. Pulse rates rise normally during excitement, following physical exertion, and during digestion.
2. The pulse rate is generally more rapid in females.
3. The pulse rate is also influenced by the breathing rate.
4. Variation of one degree of temperature above 98° F. is approximately equivalent to a rise of 10 beats in pulse

rate. *See also* Temperature—Pulse Relations.

5. Irregularity of the pulse may signify a heart condition.

6. Too slow a pulse is as important as too rapid a pulse.

7. Innumerable disorders, illnesses, and conditions cause variation from the normal pulse rate. They are too numerous to list here.

IV. Respiration: Normal Breathing Rates

Age	Number of Respirations per Minute
First year	25 to 35
12th to 17th year	20 to 25
Adulthood	16 to 18

1. Breathing rates rise normally during excitement, following physical exertion,

and, slightly, when talking rapidly and
during digestion.
2. Breathing rates are lowest at rest and
during sleep.
3. Breathing rates tend to rise with the
pulse rate.

V. Drug Doses*

Liquids

Apothecary doses	Metric System doses

---

1 quart	1000 cc.†
1 pint	500 cc.
8 fluid ounces	240 cc.
3 1/2 fluid ounces	100 cc.
1 fluid ounce	30 cc.
4 fluid drams	15 cc.
1 fluid dram	4 cc.
15 minims (drops)	1 cc.
1 minim (drop)	0.06 cc.

*All equivalents are approximate.
†A cubic centimeter (cc.) is 1/1000 of a liter.

1 teaspoonful is approximately 5 cc., or 1/6 ounce

6 teaspoonsful are approximately 30 cc., or 1 ounce

3 teaspoonsful are approximately equal to 1 tablespoonsful

Solids

Apothecary doses	Metric System doses
1 ounce	30 grams
4 drams	15 grams
1 dram	4 grams
60 grains (1 dram)	4 grams
30 grains (1/2 dram)	2 grams
15 grains	1 gram
10 grains	0.6 grams
1 grain	60 milligrams (mg.)
3/4 grain	50 mg.
1/2 grain	30 mg.
1/4 grain	15 mg.
1/6 grain	10 mg.
1/10 grain	6 mg.
1/100 grain	0.6 mg.

Doses

VI. The Home Medicine Chest

1. Contents (Medical Supplies)

Adhesive bandages, 1 box
Adhesive tape, 1 roll of 1 inch
    1 roll of 2 inch
Alcohol, 1 bottle of rubbing (70 percent alcohol, to be used as a skin antiseptic instead of iodine, etc.)
Applicators, 1 dozen with cotton tips
Bandages, 1 roll of 1-inch-wide gauze
    1 roll of 2-inch-wide gauze
    1 three-inch wide (Ace semi-elastic)
Bedpan
Bell (so patient may summon aid, if necessary)
Cotton, 1 large roll of sterile
Douche bag and attachments
Electric pad
Enamel basin (for preparing wet dressing; for bathing patient, etc.)
Enema bag and attachments
Flashlight
Gauze pads, 1 dozen sterile (paper-wrapped)
    2 x 2 inch
    1 dozen sterile (paper-wrapped)
    4 x 4 inch
Glass drinking tube

Hydrogen peroxide, 1 bottle (for use as a skin
    antiseptic)
Ice bag
Rubber pad (to go under sheets or to be used
    when wet dressings are being applied)
Rubber tubing, 1 two-foot-length (for possi-
    ble use as a tourniquet)
Scissors, 1 pair (preferably bandage scissors)
Steam inhalator and electrical attachments
Thermometers, 1 mouth
    1 rectal
Tweezers, 1 pair (for splinter removal)
Urinal
Vaseline, 1 tube or bottle of sterile

2. Medicines*

Aspirin tablets, 1 botle of 5 grain
Bicarbonate of soda, 1 box of powdered
Bicarbonate of soda tablets, 1 bottle of 10
    grain
Boric acid, 1 box of powdered

*Please note that powerful medications such as strong sleeping
tablets, narcotics, strong antiseptics such as iodine, and other special
medications are *purposely* omitted from this list. Such drugs should be
kept apart from the family medicine chest.

Collyrium eyewash with eyecup, 1 bottle
Epsom salts, 1 box of powdered
Milk of magnesia, 1 bottle
Paregoric, 1 ounce bottle
Salt tablets, 1 bottle of 5 grain
Sodium perborate powder, 1 container (for mouth wash)
Talcum powder, 1 container of any bland type
Tincture of benzoin, 1 bottle
Witch hazel, 1 bottle

3. Precautions

1. Every medication and bottle must be clearly labeled.

2. If label is not easily read, throw medication away.

3. *All* medications, no matter how mild, must be kept out of children's reach!

4. Read every label *twice* before giving medication.

5. Any poison, or special medication, should be under lock and key. Do *not* keep such medications in your regular medicine cabinet where the whole family may get to them.

6. When in doubt as to the freshness of a medicine, throw it away.

7. Do *not* ever take a medication in the dark.

8. *Never* apply a hot, wet dressing unless it has been tested for intensity of heat by the patient himself. It is better too cool than too hot.

9. Do *not* go to sleep with an electric pad turned on.

10. Do *not* keep an icebag in place more than 1/2 hour at a time.

VII. CONTAGIOUS DISEASES

Disease	Cause	How Transmitted	When Contagious?	Symptoms
Roseola (Exanthem Subitum)	Virus	Not definitely known.	Not known.	Fever for 3 days followed by rash and swollen glands.
Mumps (Parotitis)	Virus	By direct contact, coughing, sneezing, etc.	As long as swelling of glands lasts.	Fever, pain and swelling of face and under the jaw.
Measles (Rubeola)	Virus	By direct contact, coughing, sneezing, etc.	A day before rash and throughout its appearance.	Fever, running nose and eyes, Koplik spots, cough, rash.
German measles (Rubella)	Virus	By direct contact, coughing, sneezing, etc.	2 days before and 3 days after rash appears.	Fever, symptoms of cold, enlarged glands in back of neck, rash.
Chicken-pox (Varicella)	Virus	By direct contact, coughing, sneezing etc.	A day before appearance of rash and 6 days after.	Fever, pock rash, scabs, itching.

Rash Characteristics	Possible Complications	Treatment	Is Quarantine Necessary?	Is 2nd Attack Possible?
Looks like mild measles. Rash all over body.	Very rarely, convulsions.	None usually required.	No	No
None	Inflammation of testicles, ovaries, pancreas, encephalitis.	Rest in bed, medicine to relieve fever and pain.	Yes, while swelling of glands persists.	No
Starts on head, extends on to body. Purplish red spots.	Ear and gland inflammation, pneumonia, encephalitis.	Cough mixture, medicine to reduce fever, sponging.	Yes, until rash disappears.	No
Appears as a light, mild measles rash.	None	None usually required.	No	No
Individual blisters, scabs, crusts over face and body.	Occasional pneumonia, rarely encephalitis.	None usually, except to relieve fever and itching.	No	No

Disease	Cause	How Transmitted	When Contagious?	Symptons
Whooping cough *(Pertussis)*	Pertussis Bacillus	By direct contact, coughing, sneezing, etc.	During coughing spells: usually about 4 weeks.	Onset like that of cold then characteristic cough develops.
Scarlet fever *(Scarlatina)*	Streptococcus	By direct contact, contaminated milk, clothing.	From onset of symptoms and a week thereafter.	Fever, sore throat, headache, vomiting, and characteristic rash.
Polio-myelitis *(Infantile paralysis)*	Polio Virus Types I, II, III.	By direct contact, possibly through food or water.	2 days before onset and 4—6 weeks thereafter.	Fever, headache, vomiting, sore throat, diarrhea, stiff neck, pains paralysis.
Diphtheria	Diphtheria Bacillus	Contact with patient or carrier.	From onset of symptoms and 2 weeks thereafter	Fever, sore throat, characteristic membrane in throat.

Rash Charac- teristics	Possible Complica- tions	Treatment	Is Quarantine Necessary?	Is 2nd Attack Possible?
None	Pneumonia, encepha- litis.	Antibiotic drugs and injections of immune serum.	Yes, for about 4 weeks.	No
Pinpoint scarlet rash on body; little or none on face.	Inflammation of ears, glands, kidneys, rheumatic fever.	Penicillin or other antibiotic drugs.	Yes, for 7—10 days.	No
None	Brain in- volvement (Bulbar). Paralysis of respira- tion etc.	Respirator, if neces- sary. Or- thopedic care for paralysis.	Yes, 1 month.	Each type conveys its own perma- nent im- munity.
None	Inflammation of heart muscle, paralysis of palate, neuritis.	Diphtheria antitoxin, antibiotics.	Yes, until throat cultures are normal.	Yes, unless booster shots are given.

Incub

INCUBATION PERIODS

(The interval of time between exposure to disease
and development of symptoms)

Disease	Incubation Period
Amebic dysentery	3—6 days
Chickenpox (Varicella)	14—21 days
Cholera	2—3 days
Common cold	1—3 days
Diphtheria	2—5 days
Encephalitis (Epidemic encephalitis)	Probably 3—7 days
German Measles (Rubella)	14—21 days
Gonorrhea	4—7 days
Grippe	1—3 days
Infectious Hepatitis (Catarrhal Jaundice)	2—6 weeks
Infectious mononucleosis (Glandular fever)	5—15 days
Influenza	1—3 days
Leprosy	Several months-several years
Malaria	5—10 days
Malta fever (Undulant fever, Brucellosis)	2 weeks-several months
Measles (Rubeola)	10—14 days

Disease	Incubation Period
Meningitis (Epidemic meningitis)	2—4 days
Mumps (Epidemic parotitis)	12—24 days
Paratyphoid fever (Salmonella fever)	2—5 days
Plague (Bubonic plague)	3—8 days
Pneumonia (Lobar pneumonia)	2—4 days
Poliomyelitis (Infantile paralysis)	7—14 days
Rabies (Hydrophobia)	10 days—2 years
Rocky Mountain Spotted Fever (Rickettsial disease)	3—7 days
Roseola (Exanthem subitum)	7—17 days
Salmonella (Paratyphoid fever)	2—5 days
Scarlet fever (Scarlatina)	3—6 days
Smallpox	10—14 days
Syphilis (Lues)	20—30 days
Tetanus (Lockjaw)	5—10 days
Typhoid fever	10—14 days
Typhus fever	7—14 days
Whooping cough (Pertussis)	7—10 days
Yellow fever	3—6 days

VII. IMMUNIZATION AND VACCINATION TABLES

Disease	Material used	When given	Number of injections	Spacing of injections
Diph-theria	Diphtheria toxoid	Infancy and childhood, or on exposure	3	1 month
Whoop-ing cough	Pertussis vaccine	Infancy and childhood, or on exposure	3	1 month
Tetanus	Tetanus toxoid	Infancy and childhood, or after injury	3	1 month
Smallpox	Cowpox virus	Infancy, child-hood, and adulthood	1	....
Polio-myelitis	Salk polio vaccine	Infancy to 40 years or older	3—4	First two 1 month apart, third 7 months later
	Sabin polio vaccine	3, 4, 5 months of age	No, injec-tions, 3 oral doses	1 month

Reactions	Duration of immunity	Recall or booster injections	Remarks
None to slight	Varies	1st booster-after 1 year; 2d and 3rd-2-year intervals; 4th and 5th—3-year intervals and on exposure to disease	All three (diphtheria, tetanus, and whooping cough) may be combined in a single injection (in young children only)
Slight to moderate	Varies		
None to slight	Varies		
Moderate	Several years	5—7 years and for foreign travel	....
None	Unknown (probably long)	4th injection one year after 3d injection	Now used only occasionally
None	Probably permanent	Not necessary	....

Disease	Material used	When given	Number of injections	Spacing of injections
Typhoid fever	Typhoid, paratyphoid vaccine	When traveling to suspicious area	3	1—4 weeks
Mumps	Mumps vaccine	During adolescence or adulthood	2	1 week
Infectious Hepatitis	Gamma globulin	On exposure to case of infectious hepatitis	1	....
Scarlet fever	Penicillin	On exposure to case of scarlet fever	3	Daily
Rabies	Rabies vaccine	Following suspicious animal bite	14	Daily
Cholera	Cholera vaccine	When traveling to suspicious area	2	7—10 days
Typhus fever	Typhus vaccine	When traveling to suspicious area	2—3	1 week

Reactions	Duration of immunity	Recall or booster injections	Remarks
Moderate	1—3 years	Every 1—3 years	....
Bad if sensitive to eggs	Unknown	None	Not given to those sensitive to eggs
None	4—6 weeks	None	....
None	4—6 weeks	Same procedure if reexposed	May give penicillin only in adequate dosage
Slight	3—6 months	If bitten again after 3 months	May not need full series if animal is found not infected
Slight	Short	Every 6—12 months	....
Slight	Short	Every 12 months	....

Disease	Material Used	When given	Number of injections	Spacing of injections
Yellow fever	Yellow fever vaccine	When traveling to suspicious area	1	....
Plague	Plague vaccine	When traveling to suspicious area	2—3	1 week
Influenza	Influenza vaccine	During epidemics	2	1 week
Rocky Mountain spotted fever	Rocky Mountain spotted fever vaccine	When exposed to ticks in suspicious areas	3	1 week
Measles	Measles vaccine	9 to 12 months of age	3	1 month
German measles	German measles virus	Childhood; adulthood for females of childbearing age	1	....
Chicken-pox	None			

Reactions	Duration of immunity	Recall or booster injections	Remarks
May be moderate	Long	Every 6 years	Must be careful of reactions in those sensitive to eggs
Slight	Short	Every 6—12 months	....
Slight	Short	....	....
Moderate	Short	Annually	Must be careful of reactions in those sensitive to eggs
Moderate	Long	None	....
None	Unknown (probably long)	None	Woman should not be pregnant, nor become pregnant for 2 months

XI. IMPORTANT ORGANS OF THE BODY

Name of Organ	Location	Major Function
Adenoids	High up in back of throat behind nose.	Unknown. (They frequently are enlarged in children and obstruct nasal breathing.)
Adrenal glands (*Suprarenal*)	Located just above kidneys in loin.	Essential to life and for hormone secretions such as adrelanin, cortisone, etc. Regulates chemistry of essential body chemicals such as sodium, chlorides, potassium.
Anus	Outlet of intestinal tract.	Its muscles control bowel evacuation.
Appendix	In right lower part of abdomen, near beginning of large intestine.	None. (It is a vestige of man's primitive past.)
Bladder (*Urinary*)	In lower abdomen, in midline above pubic bones.	Acts as reservoir for urine which has been excreted by kidneys.

Name of Organ	Location	Major Funciton
Bone marrow	Inside of bones.	Manufactures blood cells.
Brain	Within the skull.	Control of mental and nerve activities.
a. Cerebrum	Upper portion of brain.	Higher brain functions, such as thought processes, movements, etc.
b. Cerebellum	Below cerebrum.	Controls muscle reflexes, equilibrium, etc.
c. Pons	Below cerebellum, at base of brain.	Receives and transmits impulses from cerebrum.
d. Medulla *(medulla oblongata)*	Below pons extending to spinal cord.	Transmits impulses received from higher brain centers.
Bronchial tubes	In chest, extending from trachea (windpipe) into lungs.	These are the tubes through which air moves in and out of the lungs.

Name of Organ	Location	Major Function
Breasts	Chest wall.	Female: To secrete milk. Male: None.
Cervix of Uterus	In vagina; lower-most portion of uterus.	Acts as barrier to infection; acts as passageway for sperm to enter uterus; dilates at childbirth to allow exit of unborn child.
Colon	In abdomen.	Absorbs water from stool; propels stool on toward anus.
a. Cecum	In right lower part of abdomen, connecting with small intestine.	
b. Ascending	Extends up right side of abdomen, from cecum to transverse colon.	

Name of Organ	Location	Major Function
c. Transverse	Across abdomen from ascending to descending colon.	
d. Descending	Down left side of abdomen to sigmoid colon.	
e. Sigmold	In left lower part of abdomen, from descending colon down to rectum.	
f. Rectum	In pelvis extending from sigmoid colon down to anus.	
g. Anus	Last inch of bowel.	

Name of Organ	Location	Major Function
Duode-num	In upper midabdomen, extending for 8—10 inches from stomach to jejunum (part of small intestine).	Receives food from stomach and propels it on; receives bile from liver and gallbladder; receives digestive juices from pancreas; secretes digestive juices of its own.
Esophagus *(foodpipe)*	Extending from throat to stomach.	Transports swallowed food to stomach.
Fallopian tubes *(uterine tubes)*	Extend outward from uterus for 3—4 inches to ovaries.	Transports egg from ovary to uterus. Fertilization of egg takes place within fallopian tube.
Gallbladder	In upper right part of abdomen beneath ribs.	Stores and concentrates bile received from liver, and expels it into bile ducts, which carry it to intestinal tract.
Heart	In chest, extending slightly to right of midline, but mostly to left of midline.	Pumps blood throughout body.

Name of Organ	Location	Major Function
Ileum	In midabdomen, extending from jejunum to cecum (large intestine) in right lower part of abdomen.	Absorbs food; absorbs water from intestinal contents; aids in digesting foods; propels contents on to large intestine.
Jejunum	In midabdomen, extending from duodenum down to ileum.	Absorbs food; absorbs water from intestinal contents; aids in digesting foods; propels contents onward.
Kidneys	In back, on both sides, below level of ribs in loins	Filters, excretes, and reabsorbs and thus helps to control balance of blood constituents.
Larynx	In neck, behind Adam's apple.	Controls act of speaking.
Liver	In abdomen, beneath diaphragm, more on right than on left.	Manufactures bile, controls metabolism of proteins, stores fat and sugar, and purifies the blood.

Name of Organ	Location	Major Function
Lungs	In both sides of chest cavity.	Lungs are the organs of respiration. They extract oxygen from air which is inhaled and they get rid of carbon dioxide with air which is exhaled.
Ovaries	In pelvis, on each side of uterus, adjacent to fallopian tubes.	Produce an egg each month which, when fertilized, forms an embryo. Manufacture female hormones which are secreted into blood stream.
Pancreas	In upper midabdomen just below level of stomach, near duodenum.	Manufactures insulin, which controls sugar metabolism. Manufactures juices which help to digest foods.
Parathyroid glands	Four small glands located behind thyroid in neck.	Manufacture a hormone which controls metabolism of calcium and phosphorus. (Their removal may lead to convulsions and eventual death.)
Penis	In genital region, below pubis.	Male organ of intercourse; also acts as conveyor of urine from bladder.

Name of Organ	Location	Major function
Pharynx	Behind nose and mouth.	Commonly called the throat, it is the passageway for food and drink and also for air which is breathed.
Pituitary gland	At base of skull in a hollowed-out place in the bone (the sella turcica.)	A most important gland whose hormone secretions, directly or indirectly, control metabolism. It is responsible for growth and for proper thyroid, adrenal, and ovarian gland function.
Prostate gland	Located around bladder outlet in males.	It secretes fluid in which sperm are transported during ejaculation.
Pylorus	That part of stomach adjacent to duodenum.	Its strong muscle fibers regulate outflow of stomach contents into duodenum (beginning of small intestine.)
Rectum	In pelvis; the continuation of descending and sigmoid colon.	It conveys stool toward outlet of intestinal tract.
Seminal vesicles	Located just above prostate gland in male pelvis.	Store semen for discharge through the ejaculatory ducts when orgasm takes place.

Name of Organ	Location	Major Function
Spinal cord	Within spinal canal of vertebral column, extending from base of brain to the lower back region.	This structure contains the nerves which travel from and to the brain and thus are responsible for sensation and movements.
Spleen	In upper left part of abdomen, just beneath diaphragm.	In the unborn child, it manufactures blood cells. In the fully formed human, it destroys old, worn-out blood cells.
Stomach	In left upper part of abdomen.	It churns undigested food and initiates digestion. It manufactures hydrochloric acid which helps to break down large food particles.
Testicles	Below penis in scrotal sac.	They manufacture sperm which are conveyed by the vas deferens to the penis. They secrete male hormone into blood stream.
Thymus gland	In upper front part of chest, beneath breastbone.	Its function is not known. After the second year of life it degenerates.
Thyroid gland	On both sides of trachea (windpipe) in front of neck.	Manufactures the hormone, thyroxin which controls metabolism.

Name of Organ	Location	Major Function
Tongue	Occupies floor of the mouth.	An organ of taste; assists chewing and swallowing; aids in the act of speaking.
Tonsils	On boths sides of the mouth, behind tongue.	Functions unknown. (Some think it is helpful in preventing bacteria from entering the body.)
Trachea (windpipe)	Extends from larynx in neck to bronchial tubes in chest.	Conveys air into and out of lungs.
Ureters	Extend from kidneys to bladder, behind abdominal organs.	Conveys urine from kidneys to bladder.
Urethra	A tube extending from bladder to outside. In male, it courses through penis. In female, it is located just above vaginal opening.	Conveys urine from bladder to outside.
Uterus	In pelvis just behind bladder and in front of rectum.	The organ (the womb) within which the embryo develops.
Vagina	The membranous canal located in front of rectum and below urethra.	The female organ of intercourse leading to the cervix (entrance to the uterus.) It is also through this canal that the newborn child is delivered.

PLEASE WRITE DOWN THE NUMBERS YOU MAY NEED . . . IN CASE OF AN EMERGENCY.

FIRE
POLICE
AMBULANCE
DOCTOR, HOME
DOCTOR, OFFICE

Remember, too, your Operator is available in case of emergency. Simply dial "O" (Operator) for assistance. If you cannot stay at the telephone, tell the Operator the exact location where help is needed.